Ashley Fitzgerald

SOMATIC THERAPY
101 EXERCISES FOR BODY RECONNECTION

Published by UNITEXTO

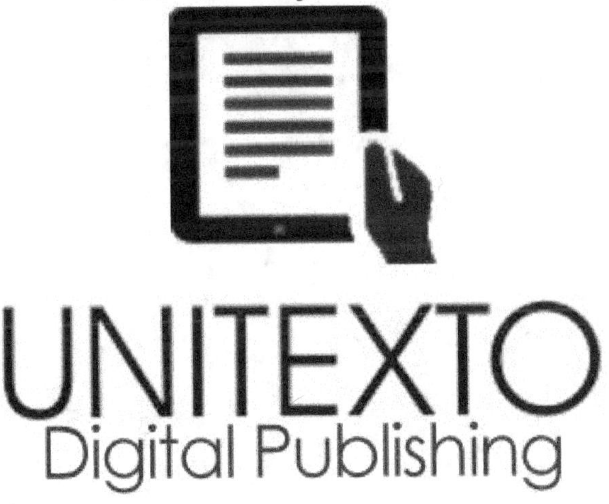

TABLE OF CONTENTS

Practices that enhance body awareness and presence through focused attention and mental exercises.

Why This Book?

In a world increasingly dominated by technology and rapid pace, it's easy to become disconnected from our own bodies. Modern lifestyles often lead to stress, anxiety, and a sense of disconnection from our physical selves. "Somatic Therapy: 101 Exercises for Body Reconnection" addresses this growing concern by providing a comprehensive guide to restoring the mind-body connection through a variety of somatic exercises.

Somatic therapy is based on the idea that the body holds onto stress and trauma, and that by engaging in specific physical practices, individuals can release these stored tensions. The benefits of somatic therapy are well-documented, offering a holistic approach to mental and physical health. This book is essential for anyone seeking to enhance their well-being through a deeper understanding of the mind-body connection.

One of the primary reasons to choose this book is its breadth of content. It covers a wide range of techniques, each designed to address different aspects of bodily awareness and emotional health. From breathwork to grounding exercises, body scanning, movement exercises, touch and massage, mindfulness and meditation, somatic experiencing, expressive arts, progressive muscle relaxation, and vocalization exercises, this book provides a comprehensive toolkit for anyone looking to improve their somatic awareness.

Breathwork, for example, is a fundamental aspect of somatic therapy. It involves various breathing techniques that promote relaxation, reduce stress, and increase awareness of bodily sensations. By focusing on the breath, individuals can calm their nervous systems and create a sense of inner peace. Techniques such as diaphragmatic breathing, alternate nostril breathing, and deep belly breathing are explored in detail, providing practical tools for managing stress and anxiety.

Grounding exercises are another crucial component of somatic therapy. These techniques help individuals feel more connected to the present moment and their physical bodies. Grounding can be as simple as feeling the weight of one's body against a chair or focusing on the sensation of feet touching the ground. These exercises are particularly useful for managing dissociation, a common symptom of trauma and anxiety. By reconnecting with the physical sensations of the body, individuals can anchor themselves in the present and reduce the impact of distressing thoughts and emotions.

Body scanning involves paying close attention to different parts of the body to notice and release tension or stored emotions. This technique helps individuals become more aware of where they hold tension and provides a method for consciously relaxing these areas. Body scanning can be particularly beneficial for those who experience chronic pain or stress-related physical symptoms.

Movement exercises encourage spontaneous or structured movement to release physical tension and improve emotional expression. Activities like dancing, stretching, or practicing yoga can help individuals express emotions that may be difficult to articulate verbally. Movement can also enhance physical health by improving flexibility, strength, and overall bodily coordination.

Touch and massage techniques are used to release tension and promote relaxation. Gentle touch can be profoundly healing, helping to soothe the nervous system and foster a sense of safety and comfort. This book explores various massage techniques and the benefits of therapeutic touch, making it accessible even to those without prior experience in massage therapy.

Mindfulness and meditation practices are integral to somatic therapy, enhancing body awareness and presence through focused attention and mental exercises. These practices help individuals cultivate a non-judgmental awareness of their bodily sensations, thoughts, and emotions. Techniques such as body scan meditation, mindfulness of breath, and loving-kindness meditation are discussed in detail.

Somatic experiencing is a therapeutic approach that helps individuals process trauma by slowly and safely revisiting traumatic memories and focusing on bodily sensations. This method, developed by Peter Levine, is designed to release the energy trapped in the body due to trauma, allowing individuals to heal from their traumatic experiences gradually and safely.

Expressive arts incorporate art, music, or drama to facilitate the expression of emotions and experiences through creative outlets. These activities provide a non-verbal way to process and express complex emotions, making them especially beneficial for those who find it challenging to articulate their feelings.

Progressive muscle relaxation (PMR) involves systematically tensing and then relaxing different muscle groups in the body to reduce physical tension and promote overall relaxation. This technique is effective in managing stress and anxiety and can be easily integrated into daily routines.

Vocalization exercises encourage the use of the voice, such as humming, chanting, or making specific sounds, to help release emotional tension and improve emotional expression. These exercises can be particularly empowering, helping individuals to express themselves more freely and confidently.

"Somatic Therapy: 100 Exercises for Body Reconnection" is an invaluable resource for anyone looking to reconnect with their bodies and improve their overall well-being. By offering a wide range of exercises and techniques, this book provides practical tools for managing stress, healing from trauma, and fostering a deeper connection between mind and body. Whether you are a therapist, a practitioner of somatic techniques, or simply someone looking to enhance your well-being, this book will serve as a comprehensive guide on your journey to body reconnection.

Ashley Fitzgerald

About the Author:

Ashley Fitzgerald: An Embodiment of Healing and Personal Triumph

From a tender age, I, Ashley Fitzgerald, was acutely attuned to the nuances of health and personal well-being. These early inklings of self-awareness were not just passing contemplations but the seeds of a lifelong journey towards self-improvement and healing.

As the chapters of life unfolded, I embraced my calling with fervor, transforming my youthful concerns into a robust career that spans two decades. Today, I stand before you not merely as a practitioner but as a seasoned professional healer whose hands and heart have been instrumental in guiding countless individuals towards weight loss triumphs, enriched sexual health, and the surmounting of life's multifaceted challenges to reach the pinnacle of their health aspirations.

My professional and academic journey is a tapestry of diverse yet interconnected disciplines. With an insatiable thirst for knowledge, I delved deep into the realms of yoga and meditation, not just as practices but as academic pursuits, seeking to understand their profound effects on the human psyche and physiology.

This spiritual and intellectual quest further led me to the healing energies of Reiki, the organic wisdom in health foods, and the transformative potential of neuroscience and positive psychology. My foray into the science of health and exercise is not merely academic; it is a reflection of my intrinsic philosophy that the body and mind are inextricable partners in the dance of life.

My dedication to personal growth extends beyond my professional endeavors—it is a way of life. Each morning, as the world stirs awake, I find sanctuary in my daily rituals. My practice of yoga is more than a physical regimen; it is a journey towards achieving a state of zen-like tranquility, a testament to my belief in the power of simplicity and inner peace. Meditation accompanies yoga as my mental compass, guiding me through life's tumultuous waves with a steadfast calm.

What fuels my unyielding passion is an unwavering drive—an innate desire to not only absorb the myriad teachings that life has to offer but also to disseminate them. I am imbued with a relentless drive to unearth and share life strategies that spark a transformative flame within souls, urging them to reach for health, well-being, and the fruition of their deepest dreams.

It was this very desire that led me to the world of writing, to become a scribe of my experiences and insights. My pen is driven by a profound commitment to be a beacon of positivity, influencing the lives of others through words that resonate with truth and vitality.

As you turn the pages of my books, what you will find is a reflection of my heart's work. I invite you into my world, not just as a reader, but as a fellow traveler on this grand adventure of life. Thank you for embarking on this journey with me, and it is my sincerest hope that you will find as much joy in reading my writings as I found in penning them down. May the words you peruse inspire you to cultivate the health and happiness you so richly deserve.

Chapter 1. Breathwork:

Focuses on various breathing techniques to promote relaxation, reduce stress, and increase awareness of bodily sensations

1. Breath Awareness Meditation

- Description:
Sit comfortably with your eyes closed. Focus on your breath as it enters and leaves your nostrils. Notice the sensation of the air, its temperature, and the rhythm of your breathing without trying to change it.

- Precautions:
Ensure you are in a quiet, comfortable space where you won't be disturbed. Avoid if you have respiratory issues.

- Goals:
To increase mindfulness and awareness of bodily sensations.

- Final State:
 A relaxed state with heightened awareness of your body's natural rhythms.

2. Deep Diaphragmatic Breathing:

- Description:
Lie on your back with knees bent. Place one hand on your chest and the other on your abdomen. Inhale deeply through your nose, allowing your abdomen to rise, then exhale slowly through your mouth.

- Precautions:

Perform in a safe environment to avoid dizziness or hyperventilation.

- Goals:
To promote relaxation and reduce stress.

- Final State:
A sense of calm and reduced tension.

3. Box Breathing:
- Description:
Inhale deeply for a count of four, hold the breath for four, exhale for four, and hold again for four. Repeat several times.

- Precautions:
Start with shorter holds if new to breathwork to avoid light-headedness.

- Goals: To enhance focus and reduce anxiety.

- Final State: Improved concentration and a sense of groundedness.

4. Alternate Nostril Breathing:

- Description:
Sit comfortably and close your right nostril with your thumb. Inhale through the left nostril, close it with your ring finger, release the right nostril, and exhale. Inhale through the right nostril, close it, release the left, and exhale. Repeat.

- Precautions:
Avoid if you have nasal congestion or sinus issues.

- Goals:
To balance the nervous system and promote mental clarity.

- Final State:
A balanced and harmonized energy flow.

5. 4-7-8 Breathing:

- Description:
Inhale through your nose for four counts, hold for seven counts, and exhale through your mouth for eight counts. Repeat several cycles.

- Precautions:
Practice sitting or lying down to prevent dizziness.

- Goals:

To calm the mind and prepare for sleep.
- Final State:
A state of deep relaxation and readiness for restful sleep.

6. Breath Counting:

- Description: Sit comfortably and count each breath, from one to ten, and then start over. If your mind wanders, gently bring your focus back to counting.

- Precautions:
Maintain a comfortable and relaxed posture.

- Goals:

To improve focus and mindfulness.

- Final State:
Increased mental clarity and presence.

7. Humming Bee Breath (Bhramari):

- Description:
Sit comfortably, close your eyes, and take a deep breath in. While exhaling, make a humming sound like a bee. Feel the vibrations in your head and chest.

- Precautions:
Avoid if you have severe throat or ear issues.

- Goals:
To reduce anxiety and enhance concentration.

- Final State:
A calm and focused mind with reduced stress levels.

8. Resonant or Coherent Breathing:

- Description:
Inhale and exhale for the same count, typically five to six seconds each. Find a rhythm that feels comfortable and maintain it.

- Precautions:
Do not force the breath; keep it natural and relaxed.

- Goals:
To promote heart rate variability and overall well-being.

- Final State:
A balanced and harmonious physiological state.

9. Lions Breath:

- Description:
Sit or kneel comfortably, inhale deeply through your nose, then open your mouth wide and stick out your tongue while exhaling forcefully with a "ha" sound.

- Precautions:
Perform in a comfortable and private setting.

- Goals:
To relieve tension and stimulate the throat chakra.

- Final State:
A sense of release and revitalization.

10.Equal Breathing (Sama Vritti):

- Description:
Inhale for a count of four, and exhale for a count of four, ensuring the breath length is equal. Repeat for several cycles.

- Precautions:
Practice gently, without straining your breath.

- Goals:
To create balance and reduce stress.

- Final State:
A balanced and peaceful state of mind and body.

These exercises aim to help individuals develop a deeper awareness of their bodies and emotions by using various breathing techniques. Each exercise has specific goals, such as promoting relaxation, reducing stress, enhancing focus, and improving overall well-being. The final state achieved through these exercises is generally one of calm, balance, and increased mindfulness.

Chapter 2. Grounding Exercises:

Techniques that help individuals feel more connected to the present moment and their physical body. Examples include feeling the weight of one's body against a chair or focusing on the sensation of feet touching the ground.

1. Body Scan:

- Description:
Lie down or sit comfortably. Slowly direct your attention to each part of your body, starting from the toes up to the head, noticing any sensations.

- Precautions:
Ensure a comfortable and quiet environment to avoid distractions.

- Goals:
To enhance body awareness and relaxation.

- Final State:
A heightened sense of bodily awareness and relaxation.

2.5-4-3-2-1 Technique:

- Description:
Identify five things you can see, four you can touch, three you can hear, two you can smell, and one you can taste.

- Precautions:
Practice in a safe and familiar environment.

- Goals:
To ground oneself in the present moment.

 - Final State:
Increased awareness of the immediate surroundings and reduced
anxiety.

3. Mindful Walking:

 - Description:
Walk slowly and deliberately, paying attention to the sensation of each step and the feeling of the ground beneath your feet.

 - Precautions:
Choose a safe and quiet path to walk.

 - Goals:
To connect with the present moment through physical movement
.

 - Final State:
A sense of calm and connection to the body.

4. Grounding Object:

 - Description:
Hold an object, such as a stone or a piece of fabric, and focus on its texture, weight, and temperature.

 - Precautions:
Select an object that is safe and comfortable to hold.

 - Goals:
To shift focus away from distressing thoughts to a physical sensation.

- Final State:
A calming and focused state of mind.

5. Feel Your Feet:

- Description:
Sit or stand and place your feet flat on the ground. Pay attention to the contact between your feet and the ground, noticing the sensations.

- Precautions:
Ensure stability to prevent falls.

- Goals:
To create a sense of grounding and stability.

- Final State:
A sense of stability and presence.

6. Progressive Muscle Relaxation:

- Description:
Tense and then relax each muscle group in your body, starting from the feet and working up to the head.

- Precautions:
Avoid tensing muscles too tightly to prevent strain.

- Goals:
To release physical tension and increase bodily awareness.

- Final State:
Relaxation and reduced physical tension.

7. Temperature Change:

- Description:
Hold something cold or splash cold water on your face to bring your attention to the present.

- Precautions:
Avoid extreme temperatures that could cause discomfort.

- Goals:
To quickly ground oneself by focusing on a strong physical sensation.

- Final State:
Increased alertness and grounding.

8. Visualization:

- Description:
Imagine yourself in a calm, safe place. Focus on the details of this place, using all your senses.

- Precautions:
Choose a visualization that feels safe and comforting.

- Goals:
To create a mental refuge and reduce stress.

- Final State:
A calm and peaceful mental state.

9. Breath Focus:

- Description:
 Sit comfortably and focus on your breath, feeling the rise and fall of your chest or abdomen.

- Precautions:
Maintain a comfortable posture to avoid strain.

- Goals:
To center attention on the breath and away from distressing thoughts.

- Final State:
A calm and focused state of mind.

10. Grounding Statements:

- Description:
Repeat grounding statements to yourself, such as "I am safe" or "I am here right now."

- Precautions:
Ensure the statements are positive and reassuring.

- Goals:
To reinforce a sense of safety and presence.

- Final State:
Increased feelings of safety and groundedness.

Chapter 3. Body Scanning:

Involves paying close attention to different parts of the body to notice and release tension or stored emotions.

1. Full Body Scan:

- Description:
Lie down or sit comfortably. Close your eyes and begin by focusing on your toes, slowly moving up to your head. Notice any tension or sensations in each part of your body.

- Precautions:
Ensure a quiet, comfortable environment. Avoid if you have severe physical pain that might be exacerbated by focusing on it.

- Goals:
To develop a comprehensive awareness of bodily sensations and release tension.

- Final State:
Deep relaxation and a sense of connection with the entire body.

2. Progressive Muscle Relaxation:

- Description:
Starting from your feet, tense each muscle group for 5-10 seconds, then relax. Move sequentially up to your head.

- Precautions:
Do not tense muscles too tightly to avoid strain.

- Goals:
To identify and release muscle tension systematically.

- Final State:
Reduced physical tension and a calm mind.

3. Guided Body Scan Meditation:

- Description:
Follow a guided meditation that directs your attention to different body parts, often available through apps or online.

- Precautions:
Choose a reliable source for the guided meditation.

- Goals:
To increase mindfulness and bodily awareness with external guidance.

- Final State:
Enhanced relaxation and mental clarity.

4. Breath-Focused Body Scan:

- Description:
Combine deep breathing with body scanning by inhaling and directing your breath to each body part you focus on.

- Precautions:
Maintain steady and comfortable breathing patterns.

- Goals:
To integrate breath awareness with bodily sensations.

- Final State:
Synchronization of breath and body awareness.

5. Sensory Awareness Scan:

- Description:
Focus on sensory details such as the temperature of your skin, the texture of your clothing, and any pressure points where your body contacts surfaces.

- Precautions:
Perform in a comfortable setting with minimal distractions.

- Goals:
To heighten sensory perception and present-moment awareness.

- Final State:
A grounded and heightened sensory experience.

6. Emotional Body Scan:

- Description:
As you scan your body, notice any areas where emotions might be stored, such as tension in the chest or tightness in the stomach. Acknowledge and release these emotions.

- Precautions:

Be gentle with yourself, especially if strong emotions arise.
- Goals:

To connect physical sensations with emotional states and facilitate emotional release.

 - Final State:
 Emotional clarity and physical relaxation.

7. Mindful Stretching:
 - Description:
Incorporate gentle stretching with a focus on how each movement affects your body. Notice the stretch and release of tension in each muscle group.

 - Precautions:
Avoid overstretching to prevent injury.

 - Goals:
To enhance body awareness through movement.

 - Final State:
Increased flexibility and body awareness.

8. Walking Body Scan:

 - Description:
While walking slowly, direct your attention to how your feet touch the ground, the movement of your legs, and the swing of your arms.

 - Precautions:
Walk in a safe and quiet area.

 - Goals:
To integrate body scanning with gentle movement.

 - Final State:

A mindful and embodied walking experience.

9. Temperature Awareness:

- Description:
Use a warm or cool object (like a heating pad or ice pack) and focus on the sensations it creates on different parts of your body.

- Precautions:
Avoid extreme temperatures that could cause discomfort or injury.

- Goals:
To enhance awareness of temperature sensations.

- Final State:
Heightened sensory awareness and relaxation.

10. Focused Attention Scan:

- Description:
Choose a specific body part to focus on for an extended period, such as your hands or feet. Notice every detail and sensation in that area.

- Precautions:
Avoid focusing on areas with acute pain or discomfort.

- Goals:
To develop a deep and detailed awareness of specific body parts.

- Final State:
Enhanced mindfulness and detailed bodily awareness.

Chapter 4. Movement Exercises:

Encourages spontaneous or structured movement to release physical tension and improve emotional expression. This can include activities like dancing, stretching, or yoga.

1. Freeform Dancing:

- Description:
Put on some music and allow your body to move freely without any structured steps. Focus on expressing your emotions through movement.

- Precautions:
Ensure you have enough space to move safely. Avoid movements that strain your body.

- Goals:
To release pent-up emotions and physical tension.

- Final State:
A sense of liberation and emotional release.

2. Sun Salutations (Yoga):

- Description:
Perform a sequence of yoga poses known as Sun Salutations. This includes poses like Mountain, Forward Bend, Plank, Cobra, and Downward Dog.

- Precautions:
Practice on a non-slip surface and modify poses if you have physical limitations.

- Goals:

To stretch and strengthen the body while promoting mindfulness.

- Final State:
Increased flexibility, strength, and a calm mind.

3. Guided Stretching:

- Description:
Follow a guided stretching routine, focusing on each muscle group. Hold each stretch for 15-30 seconds.

- Precautions:
Avoid overstretching and listen to your body to prevent injury.

- Goals:
To release muscle tension and increase flexibility.
- Final State:
Relaxed muscles and improved range of motion.

4. Tai Chi:

- Description:
Practice a series of slow, flowing movements and deep breathing. Focus on the smooth transition from one posture to another.

- Precautions:
Learn from a qualified instructor to ensure proper form.

- Goals:
To improve balance, coordination, and mental clarity.

- Final State:

Enhanced balance, reduced stress, and a sense of inner peace.

5. Expressive Writing and Movement:

- Description:
Write down your feelings for a few minutes, then translate those emotions into movement. Let your body express what you've written.

- Precautions:
Find a private space where you feel comfortable expressing yourself.

- Goals:
To connect emotions with physical expression.

- Final State:
Emotional release and a deeper understanding of your feelings.

6. Walking Meditation:

- Description:
Walk slowly and mindfully, paying attention to each step and your breath. Focus on the sensation of your feet touching the ground.

- Precautions:
Choose a safe and quiet path to walk.

- Goals:
To integrate mindfulness with physical movement.

- Final State:

A sense of calm and groundedness.

7. Dance Therapy:

- Description: Participate in a structured dance therapy session led by a certified therapist. Focus on using dance to explore and express emotions.
- Precautions: Ensure the therapist is qualified and that the space is safe for movement
.

- Goals:
To use dance as a medium for emotional exploration and healing.

- Final State:
Emotional insight and physical release.

8. Qigong:

- Description:
Practice Qigong, a form of gentle exercise involving coordinated movements, breath control, and meditation.

- Precautions:
Learn from a qualified instructor to ensure proper technique.

- Goals:
To cultivate energy (Qi) and improve overall well-being.

- Final State:
Enhanced vitality and mental clarity.

9. Body Awareness through Movement:

- Description:
Engage in activities that heighten body awareness, such as Pilates or Feldenkrais
Method. Focus on precise movements and alignment.

- Precautions:
Follow a qualified instructor to avoid improper technique.

- Goals:
To improve body awareness and alignment.
- Final State: Better posture and increased body awareness.

10. Laughter Yoga:

- Description:
Combine laughter exercises with yoga breathing techniques. Participate in group sessions where laughter is initiated through playful activities.

- Precautions:
Ensure a comfortable environment and avoid forcing laughter if it feels unnatural.

- Goals:
To reduce stress and improve mood through laughter.

- Final State:
Enhanced mood and a sense of joy and relaxation.
<response>

5. Touch and Massage:

Gentle touch or massage techniques are used to release tension and promote relaxation.

1. Self-Massage for the Shoulders and Neck:

- Description:
 Use your fingers and palms to apply gentle pressure and kneading motions to your shoulders and neck. Focus on areas that feel tense.

- Precautions:
Avoid applying too much pressure to avoid muscle strain.

- Goals:
To relieve tension and stress in the shoulder and neck area.

- Final State:
 Reduced muscle tension and a sense of relaxation.

2. Foot Reflexology:

- Description:
Use your thumbs to apply pressure to different areas of your feet, working from the toes to the heel. Focus on pressure points that correspond to different body parts.

- Precautions:
Avoid if you have foot injuries or conditions that make pressure painful.

- Goals:

To stimulate nerve endings and promote relaxation throughout the body.

- Final State:
Enhanced relaxation and improved overall well-being.

3. Hand Massage:

- Description:
Apply lotion or oil and use your fingers to massage the palms, fingers, and back of the hands with circular motions.

- Precautions:
Be gentle to avoid discomfort, especially if you have arthritis or joint issues.

- Goals:
To increase circulation and reduce stress in the hands.

- Final State:
Relaxed hands and improved dexterity.

4. Facial Massage:

- Description:
Use your fingertips to gently massage your forehead, temples, cheeks, and jaw with small circular motions.

- Precautions:
Avoid areas with skin irritation or acne.

- Goals:
To relieve facial tension and promote relaxation.

- Final State:
A relaxed and refreshed facial appearance.

5. Back Massage with a Foam Roller:

- Description:
Lie on your back with a foam roller placed under your spine. Slowly roll up and down, focusing on areas of tension.

- Precautions:
Ensure proper alignment to avoid strain. Avoid if you have back injuries.

- Goals:
To release muscle tension in the back.

- Final State:
A relaxed and tension-free back.

6. Head and Scalp Massage:

- Description:
Use your fingers to gently massage your scalp in circular motions, working from the forehead to the back of the head.

- Precautions:
Be gentle to avoid pulling hair or irritating the scalp.

- Goals:
To increase blood flow and promote relaxation.

- Final State:
Reduced stress and a sense of well-being.

7. Abdominal Massage:

- Description:
Use your fingers to gently massage your abdomen in clockwise circular motions.
- Precautions:
Avoid if you have gastrointestinal issues or discomfort.

- Goals:
To promote digestion and relieve abdominal tension.

- Final State:
Improved digestion and a relaxed abdomen.

8.Partner Shoulder Massage:

- Description:
Sit comfortably and have a partner use their hands to massage your shoulders, using kneading and circular motions.

- Precautions:
Communicate with your partner to ensure pressure is comfortable.

- Goals:
To relieve shoulder tension and promote relaxation.

- Final State:
Reduced tension and improved connection with your partner.

9.Massage with Essential Oils:

- Description:

Apply diluted essential oils to the skin and use gentle massage techniques on areas of tension.

- Precautions:
Test for allergies and avoid undiluted essential oils on the skin.

- Goals:
 To enhance relaxation through the combination of touch and aromatherapy.

- Final State:
Deep relaxation and a soothing scent.

10.Self-Massage with a Tennis Ball:

- Description:
Place a tennis ball under your back, glutes, or shoulders and gently roll over it to target knots and tension.

- Precautions:
Avoid bony areas and apply gentle pressure to prevent injury.

- Goals:
To release deep muscle tension and improve mobility.

- Final State:
Reduced muscle tightness and improved range of motion.

6. Mindfulness and Meditation:

Practices that enhance body awareness and presence through focused attention and mental exercises.

1. Mindful Breathing:

- Description:
Sit or lie down comfortably. Focus on your breath as it enters and leaves your nostrils or feel the rise and fall of your chest or abdomen.

- Precautions:
Ensure a quiet environment free from distractions.

- Goals:
To develop awareness of breath and reduce stress.

- Final State:
A calm and focused mind with improved breath awareness.

2. Body Scan Meditation:

- Description:
Lie down and mentally scan your body from head to toe, noticing any sensations or tension in each part of the body.

- Precautions:
 Avoid if you have severe pain that may distract from the practice.

- Goals:
To increase body awareness and release tension.

- Final State:
Deep relaxation and heightened body awareness.

3. Loving-Kindness Meditation:

- Description:
Sit comfortably and silently repeat phrases like "May I be happy, may I be healthy" while visualizing sending love and kindness to yourself and others.

- Precautions:
Practice in a quiet and safe environment.

- Goals:
To cultivate compassion and emotional resilience.

- Final State:
Enhanced feelings of love, compassion, and connection.

4. Mindful Eating:

- Description:
Eat a meal slowly, paying attention to the taste, texture, and aroma of each bite. Notice your body's hunger and fullness cues.

- Precautions:
Avoid distractions like TV or smartphones while eating.

- Goals:
To improve digestion and foster a healthy relationship with food.

- Final State:

Increased enjoyment of food and better awareness of hunger and satiety signals.

5. Walking Meditation:

- Description:
Walk slowly and mindfully, paying attention to the sensation of each step and the contact of your feet with the ground.

- Precautions:
Choose a safe, quiet path to avoid accidents.

- Goals:
To integrate mindfulness with physical movement.

- Final State:
A sense of calm and groundedness.

6. Mindful Listening:

- Description:
Sit quietly and focus on the sounds around you without judgment or labeling. Notice the pitch, volume, and duration of each sound.

- Precautions:
Practice in a place where you won't be interrupted.

- Goals:
To enhance listening skills and present-moment awareness.

- Final State:
Improved auditory awareness and focus.

7. Guided Imagery:

- Description:
Listen to a guided meditation that takes you through a peaceful visualization, such as a walk on the beach or a forest path.

- Precautions:
Ensure you are comfortable and won't be disturbed.

- Goals:
To reduce stress and enhance mental clarity.

- Final State:
A relaxed state of mind and improved visualization skills.

8. Mindful Stretching:

- Description:
Perform gentle stretches with full attention to the sensations in your muscles and joints.
- Precautions: Avoid overstretching to prevent injury.

- Goals:
To increase flexibility and body awareness.

- Final State:
Relaxed muscles and a heightened sense of body awareness.

9. Mindfulness of Emotions:

- Description:

Sit quietly and bring your attention to your current emotions. Observe them without judgment and notice how they manifest in your body.

- Precautions:
Be gentle with yourself, especially if strong emotions arise.

- Goals:
To increase emotional awareness and regulation.

- Final State:
A better understanding of your emotional states and improved emotional regulation.

10. Mindful Journaling:

- Description:
Spend time writing about your thoughts and feelings without judgment. Focus on the present moment and your current experiences.

- Precautions:
Find a quiet place where you can write without interruptions.

- Goals:
To process emotions and enhance self-awareness.

- Final State:
Increased clarity of thoughts and emotions and a sense of relief.

Chapter 7. Somatic Experiencing:

A therapeutic approach that helps individuals process trauma by slowly and safely revisiting traumatic memories and focusing on bodily sensations.

1. Body Awareness Exercise:

- Description:
Sit or lie down comfortably. Close your eyes and bring your attention to different parts of your body, starting from your toes and moving up to your head. Notice any sensations without judgment.

- Precautions:
Ensure you are in a safe and quiet environment to avoid distractions.

- Goals:
To increase body awareness and identify areas of tension or discomfort.

- Final State:
Improved body awareness and a sense of calm.

2. Grounding Techniques:

- Description:
Sit with your feet flat on the ground. Focus on the sensation of your feet making contact with the floor. Notice the support and stability provided by the ground.

- Precautions:
Practice in a comfortable and safe environment.

- Goals:
To enhance feelings of safety and stability.

- Final State:
A grounded and centered state of mind.

3. Pendulation:

- Description:
Alternate your focus between a feeling of safety and a small amount of trauma-related sensation. Move back and forth between these two states.

- Precautions:
Work with a therapist if possible, especially for severe trauma.

- Goals:
To build resilience and increase tolerance for traumatic memories.

- Final State:
Greater ability to manage and integrate traumatic memories.

4. Titration:

- Description:
Focus on a very small aspect of a traumatic memory or sensation. Allow yourself to experience it in manageable amounts, gradually increasing exposure.

- Precautions:
Proceed slowly and stop if feelings become overwhelming.

- Goals:
To process trauma without becoming overwhelmed.

- Final State:
Reduced intensity of traumatic memories and sensations.

5. Self-Touch:
- Description:
Gently place your hands on different parts of your body, such as your arms, chest, or abdomen. Notice the warmth and pressure of your hands.

- Precautions:
Ensure your touch is gentle and non-invasive.

- Goals:
To promote self-soothing and body connection.

- Final State:
Enhanced sense of safety and comfort.

6. Voo Sound:

- Description:
Sit comfortably and take a deep breath. As you exhale, make a low, extended "voo" sound, feeling the vibration in your chest and abdomen.

- Precautions:
Ensure you are in a quiet environment to focus on the sound.

- Goals:
To release tension and stimulate the vagus nerve.

- Final State:

Reduced stress and a relaxed state.

7. Movement Tracking:

- Description:
Allow your body to move freely in response to internal sensations. Follow these movements without judgment or restriction.

- Precautions:
Ensure you have enough space to move safely.

- Goals:
To release stored tension and emotions through movement.

- Final State:
Increased freedom of movement and emotional release.

8. Boundary Setting:

- Description:
Practice saying "no" and setting physical boundaries with objects or imaginary scenarios. Notice how your body feels as you set these boundaries.

- Precautions:
Practice in a safe and private environment.

- Goals:
To enhance personal boundaries and sense of control.

- Final State:
Strengthened personal boundaries and empowerment.

9. Visualization:

- Description:
Imagine a safe place in your mind. Visualize yourself in this place, noticing the sights, sounds, and sensations that make it feel safe.

- Precautions:
Ensure the visualization is of a place that feels genuinely safe and comforting.

- Goals:
To create a mental refuge and reduce anxiety.

- Final State:
A sense of safety and relaxation.

10. Somatic Dialogue:

- Description:
Engage in a mental conversation with different parts of your body. Ask what they need or why they feel a certain way, and listen for the response.

- Precautions:
Approach this exercise with an open mind and without judgment.

- Goals:
To understand and address bodily sensations and emotions.
- Final State:
Improved communication with and understanding of your body.

Chapter 8. Expressive Arts:

Incorporating art, music, or drama to facilitate the expression of emotions and experiences through creative outlets.

1. Intuitive Painting:

- Description:
Use paints and brushes to create art based on your feelings without planning or judgment. Allow your emotions to guide your hand.

- Precautions:
Ensure you have a clean, protected workspace to avoid spills.

- Goals:
To express emotions and uncover subconscious thoughts.

- Final State:
Emotional release and insight into your inner state.

2. Music Improvisation:

- Description:
Use musical instruments to create spontaneous music that reflects your current emotional state. Focus on the sounds and rhythms that emerge naturally.

- Precautions:
Use instruments that you are familiar with to avoid frustration.

- Goals:

To express and process emotions through sound.

- Final State:
A sense of relief and emotional expression.

3. Drama Therapy:

- Description:
Act out scenes from your life or imagined scenarios that represent your emotional experiences. Use props and costumes to enhance the experience.

- Precautions:
Ensure a safe and private space for expressive acting.

- Goals:
To explore and express emotions through role-play.

- Final State:
 Increased emotional understanding and catharsis.

4. Collage Making:

- Description:
Create a collage using magazines, photographs, and other materials to represent your emotions or life experiences.

- Precautions:
Handle cutting tools carefully and be mindful of sharp edges.

- Goals:
To visually express complex emotions and thoughts.

- Final State:
A tangible representation of your emotional landscape.

5. Creative Writing:

- Description:
Write poems, stories, or journal entries that reflect your emotions and experiences. Focus on free expression without worrying about grammar or structure.

- Precautions:
Find a quiet space to write without interruptions.

- Goals:
To articulate and process emotions through words.

- Final State:
Emotional clarity and a sense of relief.

6. Dance Therapy:

- Description:
Use dance to express your emotions. Let your body move freely to the rhythm of the music, focusing on how each movement feels.

- Precautions:
Ensure you have enough space to move safely.

- Goals:
To release emotional and physical tension through movement.

- Final State:
Physical relaxation and emotional expression.

7. Mandala Drawing:

- Description:
Draw or color mandalas as a form of meditation and self-expression. Focus on the patterns and shapes that emerge.

- Precautions:
Use coloring materials that you are comfortable with.

- Goals:
To center the mind and express inner feelings.

- Final State:
 A sense of calm and focused creativity.

8. Storytelling:

- Description:
Share personal stories or create fictional tales that reflect your emotional experiences. You can tell these stories to others or record them.

- Precautions:
Choose a supportive audience if sharing with others.

- Goals:
To process and communicate emotions through narrative.

- Final State:
 Enhanced understanding of personal experiences and emotional release.

9. Sculpting:

- Description:
Use clay or other sculpting materials to create shapes that represent your emotions. Focus on the tactile experience of molding the material.

- Precautions:
Use non-toxic materials and ensure a clean workspace.

- Goals:
To express emotions through tactile creativity.

- Final State:
A tangible expression of your emotional state.

10. Photographic Self-Expression:

- Description: Take photographs that capture your emotional experiences. Use different angles, lighting, and subjects to convey your feelings.

- Precautions:
Handle cameras carefully and respect privacy when photographing others.
- Goals:
To capture and express emotions through visual imagery.

- Final State:
A visual representation of your emotional journey.

Chapter 9. Progressive Muscle Relaxation (PMR):

This involves systematically tensing and then relaxing different muscle groups in the body to reduce physical tension and promote overall relaxation.

1. Foot Tension and Relaxation:

- Description:
Sit or lie down comfortably. Tense the muscles in your feet by curling your toes tightly for 5-10 seconds, then slowly release the tension.

- Precautions:
Avoid straining your muscles. If you feel any pain, stop immediately.

- Goals:
To release tension in the feet and enhance relaxation.

- Final State:
Relaxed and tension-free feet.

2. Calf Muscle Relaxation:

- Description:
Tighten the muscles in your calves by pointing your toes upwards towards your head for 5-10 seconds, then slowly relax.

- Precautions:
Ensure a gentle stretch without overexertion.

- Goals:
To reduce tension in the calf muscles.

- Final State:
A sense of relaxation in the lower legs.

3. Thigh Muscle Relaxation:

- Description:
Squeeze your thigh muscles by pressing your knees together or lifting your legs slightly off the ground for 5-10 seconds, then release.

- Precautions:
Avoid excessive force to prevent strain.

- Goals:
To alleviate tension in the thigh area.

- Final State:
Relaxed thigh muscles.

4. Abdominal Muscle Relaxation:

- Description:
Tense your abdominal muscles by sucking in your stomach tightly for 5-10 seconds, then gradually relax.

- Precautions:
Perform gently to avoid discomfort.

- Goals:
To release abdominal tension and promote relaxation.

- Final State:
A relaxed and calm abdomen.

5. Hand Tension and Relaxation:

- Description:
Make a fist with your hand and squeeze tightly for 5-10 seconds, then slowly open your hand and relax.

- Precautions:
Be gentle to avoid any strain on the muscles.

- Goals:
To reduce tension in the hands.

- Final State:
Relaxed and tension-free hands.

6. Arm and Shoulder Relaxation:

- Description:
Tighten the muscles in your arms by bending your elbows and pulling your forearms towards your shoulders for 5-10 seconds, then release.

- Precautions:
Avoid overexertion, especially if you have shoulder issues.

- Goals:
To relieve tension in the arms and shoulders.

- Final State:
Relaxed arm and shoulder muscles.

7. Neck Muscle Relaxation:

- Description:

Gently tilt your head back slightly to tense your neck muscles for 5-10 seconds, then slowly bring your head back to a neutral position.

   - Precautions:
Avoid sudden or extreme movements to prevent injury.

   - Goals:
To ease tension in the neck area.

   - Final State:
A relaxed and tension-free neck.

8.   Facial Muscle Relaxation:

   - Description:
Tighten your facial muscles by scrunching your face tightly for 5-10 seconds, then slowly relax all facial muscles.

   - Precautions:
Be gentle to avoid discomfort.

   - Goals:
To release tension in the face.

   - Final State:
Relaxed and calm facial muscles.

9.   Chest and Back Relaxation:

   - Description:
Take a deep breath and expand your chest, holding the breath and tensing your chest muscles for 5-10 seconds, then slowly exhale and relax.

- Precautions:
Breathe comfortably without forcing.

- Goals:
To reduce tension in the chest and back.

- Final State:
A relaxed and tension-free chest and back.

10. Whole Body Relaxation:

- Description:
Progressively tense and relax each muscle group from your toes to your head, finishing with a full body scan to ensure all muscles are relaxed.

- Precautions:
 Perform slowly and gently, paying attention to any areas of discomfort.

- Goals:
To achieve complete physical relaxation.

- Final State:
A deeply relaxed and calm body.

Chapter10. Vocalization Exercises:

These exercises encourage the use of the voice, such as humming, chanting, or making specific sounds, to help release emotional tension and improve emotional expression.

1. Humming Meditation:

- Description: Sit comfortably and take a deep breath. As you exhale, hum a single note, feeling the vibration in your chest and head. Repeat for several minutes.
- Precautions: Ensure you are in a quiet space where you won't be disturbed.
- Goals: To promote relaxation and focus through vocal vibrations.
- Final State: A calm and centered mind with reduced tension.

2. Chanting Mantras:

- Description:
Choose a mantra or phrase that resonates with you. Sit comfortably, close your eyes, and repeat the mantra aloud in a steady rhythm.

- Precautions:
Practice in a quiet environment and choose a mantra that feels meaningful.

- Goals:
To enhance concentration and emotional grounding.

- Final State:
A sense of inner peace and emotional stability.

3. Singing Your Emotions:

- Description:
Select a song that reflects your current emotional state and sing it aloud. Focus on the emotions conveyed through the lyrics and melody.

- Precautions:
Ensure you are in a space where you feel comfortable expressing yourself.

- Goals:
To express and process emotions through music.

- Final State:
Emotional release and a feeling of catharsis.

4. Vowel Sound Meditation:

- Description:
 Sit comfortably and take a deep breath. On the exhale, vocalize a long vowel sound (e.g., "A," "E," "I," "O," "U"), focusing on the resonance in your body.

- Precautions:
Choose a quiet space to avoid interruptions.

- Goals:
To explore different resonances in the body and promote relaxation.

- Final State:
A relaxed and resonant body.

5. Toning:

- Description:
Sit or stand comfortably and produce a continuous tone at a comfortable pitch. Sustain the tone for several breaths, focusing on the sound and vibration.

- Precautions:
Avoid straining your voice by keeping the pitch comfortable.

- Goals:
To balance energy and enhance vocal awareness.

- Final State:
A sense of harmony and balanced energy.

6. Expressive Vocalization:

- Description:
Use your voice to express a range of emotions, such as joy, anger, sadness, and fear. Allow your voice to change naturally with each emotion.

- Precautions:
Practice in a private space to feel free to express all emotions.

- Goals:
To explore and release various emotions through vocal expression.

- Final State:
Emotional clarity and release.

7. Laughter Yoga:

- Description:
Engage in exercises that stimulate laughter, such as forced laughter that turns into real laughter. Focus on the sound and sensation of laughter.

- Precautions:
Practice in a safe environment and be mindful of physical limitations.

- Goals:
To reduce stress and elevate mood through laughter.

- Final State:
Increased joy and reduced stress.

8. Breath and Sound Integration:

- Description:
Combine deep breathing with vocalization. Inhale deeply and on the exhale, produce a sound like "Ahh" or "Om," extending the sound for the length of the exhale.

- Precautions:
Ensure the breath is smooth and the sound is comfortable.

- Goals:
To integrate breath and sound for relaxation and focus.

- Final State:
A calm and focused state with synchronized breath and sound.

9. Group Chanting:

- Description:
Join a group to chant together. Focus on the collective sound and the sense of connection with others.

- Precautions:
Ensure the group setting is supportive and comfortable.

- Goals:
To foster a sense of community and shared emotional experience.

- Final State:
Enhanced connection and collective emotional expression.

10.Sonic Meditation

- Description:
Use sound bowls, gongs, or other instruments to create sustained tones. Focus on the vibrations and sounds as a form of meditation.

- Precautions:
Choose instruments that are comfortable to use and produce soothing sounds.

- Goals:
To use sound vibrations to facilitate deep meditation and relaxation.

- Final State:
A deeply meditative and relaxed state.

Chapter 11. Reference books

1. The Somatic Therapy Workbook: Stress-Relieving Exercises for Strengthening the Mind-Body Connection by Livia Shapiro
   - Description: This workbook provides a range of therapist-approved activities designed to release tension, boost mood, and heal from traumatic experiences. It is an easy-to-use guide that focuses on strengthening the mind-body connection through various somatic therapy exercises.

2. Somatic Therapy Workbook - 170+ Pages of Stress-Relieving Activities and Worksheets by Livia Shapiro
   - Description: This comprehensive workbook includes over 170 pages of activities and worksheets aimed at relieving stress and promoting healing through somatic therapy techniques.

3. Waking the Tiger: Healing Trauma by Peter A. Levine
   - Description: This book explores how trauma affects the body and provides techniques for healing through somatic experiencing. Levine explains how to release trauma stored in the body to restore balance and health.

4. The Body Keeps the Score: Brain, Mind, and Body in the Healing of Trauma by Bessel van der Kolk
   - Description: Van der Kolk's seminal work explains how traumatic stress affects the body and brain. The book offers insights into various therapeutic approaches, including somatic therapies, to aid in recovery.

5. Healing Trauma: A Pioneering Program for Restoring the Wisdom of Your Body by Peter A. Levine

- Description: This guide provides practical exercises for healing trauma through somatic experiencing. Levine offers a step-by-step program to help readers reconnect with their bodies and release trauma.

6. In an Unspoken Voice: How the Body Releases Trauma and Restores Goodness by Peter A. Levine

- Description: Levine discusses the physiological and psychological effects of trauma and offers somatic exercises to help individuals release trauma and restore well-being.

7. Trauma Through a Child's Eyes: Awakening the Ordinary Miracle of Healing by Peter A. Levine and Maggie Kline

- Description: This book focuses on how trauma affects children and provides somatic techniques to help children heal from traumatic experiences.

8. Somatic Internal Family Systems Therapy: Awareness, Breath, Resonance, Movement and Touch in Practice by Susan McConnell

- Description: Integrating Internal Family Systems (IFS) with somatic therapy, this book provides exercises to address trauma and enhance emotional healing through body awareness and movement.

9. The Polyvagal Theory in Therapy: Engaging the Rhythm of Regulation by Deb Dana

- Description: Deb Dana explains the Polyvagal Theory and offers practical exercises for using this approach in therapy to help regulate the nervous system and promote healing.

10. Somatic Psychotherapy Toolbox: 125 Worksheets and Exercises for Trauma & Stress by Manuela Mischke-Reeds

- Description: This book provides a wide range of worksheets and exercises designed to help therapists and clients address trauma and stress through somatic practices.

11. The Pocket Guide to the Polyvagal Theory: The Transformative Power of Feeling Safe by Stephen W. Porges

- Description: Porges offers a concise introduction to the Polyvagal Theory and explains how it can be applied in therapeutic settings to promote safety and healing.

12. The Trauma-Sensitive Yoga Deck: 50 Practices to Calm Your Mind and Body by David Emerson

- Description: This deck of cards provides yoga practices specifically designed to help individuals recover from trauma by using somatic techniques to calm the mind and body.

13. Sensorimotor Psychotherapy: Interventions for Trauma and Attachment by Pat Ogden

- Description: Ogden's book combines somatic therapy with psychotherapy to offer interventions for trauma and attachment issues, emphasizing the importance of body awareness.

14. Somatic Experience in Depth: Psychology, Trauma, and the Body's Wisdom by Peter A. Levine and Ann Frederick

- Description: This book delves into the relationship between psychology and the body's responses to trauma, offering exercises for somatic healing.

15. The Expressive Body in Life, Art, and Therapy: Working with Movement, Metaphor, and Meaning by Daria Halprin

- Description: Halprin explores how movement and expressive arts can be used in therapy to facilitate healing and self-discovery through somatic practices.

16. Polyvagal Exercises for Safety and Connection: 50 Client-Centered Practices by Deb Dana

- Description: This book provides exercises based on the Polyvagal Theory to help clients build safety and connection through somatic practices.

17. Trauma-Sensitive Mindfulness: Practices for Safe and Transformative Healing by David A. Treleaven

- Description: Treleaven offers mindfulness practices designed to be safe and effective for individuals with trauma, integrating somatic principles.

18. The Tao of Trauma: A Practitioner's Guide for Integrating Five Element Theory and Trauma Treatment by Alaine D. Duncan and Kathy L. Kain

- Description: This book combines traditional Chinese medicine with modern trauma therapy, offering somatic exercises based on Five Element Theory.

19. The Body Remembers: The Psychophysiology of Trauma and Trauma Treatment by Babette Rothschild

- Description: Rothschild explains the connection between trauma and the body, providing exercises for trauma treatment through somatic approaches.

20. The Feldenkrais Method: Teaching by Handling by Yochanan Rywerant

- Description: This book introduces the Feldenkrais Method, which uses gentle movement and body awareness to improve physical and emotional well-being.

Chapter 12. Academic papers

1. Somatic experiencing – effectiveness and key factors of a …

- Description: This paper discusses the effectiveness of somatic experiencing in treating trauma and the key factors that contribute to its success. The study highlights how somatic exercises help in the healing process by addressing the mind-body connection.

- Source: NCBI, https://www.ncbi.nlm.nih.gov/pmc/articles/PMC8276 649/

2. What is somatic therapy?

- Description: This article from Harvard Health explores how somatic therapy helps to process deeply painful experiences by applying mind-body healing techniques. It discusses various somatic exercises and their benefits for mental health.

- Source: Harvard Health, https://www.health.harvard.edu/blog/what-is-somatic-therapy-202307072951

3. At-Home Somatic Therapy Exercises for Trauma Recovery

- Description: This paper provides practical at-home somatic therapy exercises designed for trauma recovery. It emphasizes the benefits of these exercises in managing distressing symptoms and improving mental health.

- Source: Psych Central, https://psychcentral.com/lib/somatic-therapy-exercises-for-trauma

4. Somatic Therapy: Benefits, Types And Efficacy

- Description: Published by Forbes Health, this article reviews the benefits and types of somatic therapy, including its efficacy in reducing symptoms of PTSD, depression, and anxiety through somatic exercises.
- Source: Forbes, https://www.forbes.com/health/mind/somatic-therapy/

5. Somatic Experience - Scholars Crossing

- Description: This research study explores how somatic therapy supports the mind-body connection of trauma and provides insights into its effectiveness in the healing process.
- Source: Scholars Crossing, https://digitalcommons.liberty.edu/cgi/viewcontent.cgi?article=5814&context=doctoral

6. Try These Somatic Exercises to Improve Your Mental Health

- Description: This paper discusses five specific somatic exercises and their impact on mental health, highlighting how these practices can enhance well-being and aid in the healing process.
- Source: Charlie Health, https://www.charliehealth.com/post/somatic-exercises-for-mental-health

7. Somatic Experiencing for Posttraumatic Stress Disorder: A Randomized Controlled Outcome Study

- Description: This study evaluates the effectiveness of Somatic Experiencing (SE) for treating PTSD. It showed significant improvements in symptoms and overall mental health of participants.
- Source: https://psycnet.apa.org/doi/10.1037/tra0000471

8. Somatic experiencing: Using interoception and proprioception as core elements of trauma therapy

- Description: This paper presents a theory of human trauma and chronic stress, focusing on SE techniques involving interoception, proprioception, and kinesthetic sensations to resolve trauma.
- Source: https://www.frontiersin.org/articles/10.3389/fpsyg.2018.00798/full

9. Healing the Body and Mind: Sensory and Somatic Interventions

- Description: This review explores the effectiveness of sensory and somatic interventions for interpersonal trauma, providing insights into occupational therapy practices.
- Source: https://scholarworks.indianapolis.iu.edu/bitstream/handle/1805/27003/FINAL%20RSR%20Interpersonal%20Trauma.pdf?sequence=1

10. Somatic Experiencing for Posttraumatic Stress Disorder: A Randomized Controlled Study

- Description: This randomized controlled study assesses the efficacy of SE in reducing PTSD symptoms, showing significant symptom reduction and improvement in quality of life.
- Source: https://www.academia.edu/41214607/Somatic_Experiencing_for_Posttraumatic_Stress_Disorder_A_Randomized_Controlled_Study

11. Evaluating Somatic Experiencing® to Heal Cancer Trauma: First Evidence

- Description: This paper evaluates the use of SE to address trauma in cancer patients, showing promising results in improving psychological well-being.
   - Source: https://www.mdpi.com/2077-0383/10/7/1540

12. The somatic psychotherapies | The Trauma Therapies

- Description: This chapter explores various somatic psychotherapies, including SE, and their effectiveness in treating trauma-related symptoms.
   - Source: https://academic.oup.com/book/34507/chapter/2911 71466

13. SE™ Research and Articles - Somatic Experiencing® International

- Description: This resource provides various articles and studies on the effectiveness of SE in treating trauma, PTSD, and related conditions.
   - Source: https://traumahealing.org/research/

14. How Does Somatic Experiencing Therapy Work?

- Description: This article explains the principles of SE and its application in trauma therapy, emphasizing the importance of bodily awareness and gentle processing of traumatic memories.
   - Source: https://www.verywellmind.com/how-does-somatic-experiencing-therapy-work-5187403

15. Somatic experiencing therapy: Exercises and research

- Description: This article provides an overview of SE, including exercises and research supporting its effectiveness in trauma therapy.

- Source:
https://www.medicalnewstoday.com/articles/somatic-experiencing

16. Interpersonal Neurobiology and Somatic Experiencing: Healing the Impact of Developmental Trauma

- Description: This paper discusses the integration of interpersonal neurobiology with SE to address developmental trauma, highlighting the benefits of combining these approaches.
- Source:
https://www.ncbi.nlm.nih.gov/pmc/articles/PMC5810 866/

17. The role of emotion processing in art therapy (REPAT) and somatic experiencing for trauma recovery

- Description: This study explores the efficacy of combining art therapy with SE to enhance emotional expression and trauma recovery.
- Source:
https://www.ncbi.nlm.nih.gov/pmc/articles/PMC1034 3444/

18. A Randomized Controlled Trial of Brief SE™ for Chronic Low Back Pain and Comorbid PTSD Symptoms

- Description: This trial evaluates the impact of brief SE interventions on chronic low back pain and comorbid PTSD symptoms, showing significant improvements.
- Source:
https://www.tandfonline.com/doi/full/10.1080/21642 850.2020.1843865

19. Somatic Experiencing: Enhancing Psychoanalytic Holding for Trauma and Catastrophic Dissociation

- Description: This paper discusses the integration of SE with psychoanalytic techniques to address trauma and dissociation, highlighting the complementary benefits.
- Source: https://www.tandfonline.com/doi/full/10.1080/07351690.2020.1752330

20. The Effectiveness of Somatic Experience Based Stabilization Program for Refugee Women's Post-Traumatic Stress

- Description: This study evaluates a stabilization program based on SE principles for refugee women, showing significant reductions in PTSD symptoms and improvements in mindfulness and social support.
- Source: https://www.researchgate.net/publication/351072062

21. Use of Somatic Experiencing Principles as a PTSD Prevention Tool for Children and Teens

- Description: This paper explores the application of SE principles in preventing PTSD in children and teens following acute stress events, demonstrating effectiveness in reducing symptoms.
- Source: https://www.researchgate.net/publication/348943482

22. Somatic Experiencing, EMDR, and Brainspotting: Integrative Approaches to Trauma Therapy

- Description: This study compares the efficacy of SE, EMDR, and Brainspotting in trauma therapy, highlighting the unique benefits of each approach.

- Source:
https://www.researchgate.net/publication/342828111

23. Integrating Somatic Experiencing® and Attachment into Equine-Assisted Trauma Recovery
   - Description: This paper discusses the integration of SE with equine-assisted therapy to enhance trauma recovery, showing positive outcomes in emotional regulation and attachment.
   - Source:
https://www.researchgate.net/publication/336893215

24. Somatic Experiencing and the Treatment of Chronic Pain
   - Description: This article explores the use of SE in treating chronic pain, demonstrating significant reductions in pain and improvements in overall well-being.
   - Source:
https://www.ncbi.nlm.nih.gov/pmc/articles/PMC7511744/

25. Somatic Experiencing in Family Constellations
   - Description: This study examines the application of SE in family constellation therapy, showing enhanced resolution of family trauma and improved relational dynamics.
   - Source:
https://www.researchgate.net/publication/345892134

Chapter 13. Weekly plan of activities day by day

DIABETES

Monday:
- Morning: 30-minute brisk walk
- Afternoon: Meal planning session for the week (focus on low-GI foods)
- Evening: Light stretching and relaxation exercises

Tuesday:
- Morning: 45-minute cycling session
- Afternoon: Diabetes education class (online or in-person)
- Evening: 10-minute meditation

Wednesday:
- Morning: 30-minute swimming
- Afternoon: Healthy cooking class (focus on diabetic-friendly recipes)
- Evening: Light yoga session

Thursday:
- Morning: 30-minute strength training
- Afternoon: Reading about diabetes management
- Evening: Gentle stretching exercises

Friday:
- Morning: 30-minute walk/jog
- Afternoon: Review blood sugar levels and adjust plan as needed
- Evening: Social activity with friends or family

Saturday:

- Morning: 1-hour dance class
- Afternoon: Outdoor activity (hiking, gardening)
- Evening: Light relaxation exercises

Sunday:
- Morning: 30-minute yoga session
- Afternoon: Plan meals and activities for the upcoming week
- Evening: Relax with a book or light music

HYPERTENSION

Monday:
- Morning:
  - Exercise: 30-minute brisk walk
  - Breakfast: Oatmeal with berries and nuts
- Afternoon:
  - Lunch: Grilled chicken salad with a variety of vegetables
  - Activity: 10-minute mindfulness meditation
- Evening:
  - Dinner: Baked salmon with quinoa and steamed broccoli
  - Activity: Light stretching exercises

Tuesday:
- Morning:
  - Exercise: 45-minute cycling session
  - Breakfast: Greek yogurt with honey and berries
- Afternoon:
  - Lunch: Turkey and avocado wrap with a side of mixed greens
  - Activity: 15-minute deep breathing exercises
- Evening:
  - Dinner: Vegetable stir-fry with tofu and brown rice

- Activity: Gentle yoga session

Wednesday:
- Morning:
  - Exercise: 30-minute swimming
  - Breakfast: Smoothie with spinach, banana, almond milk, and protein powder
- Afternoon:
  - Lunch: Quinoa salad with chickpeas, tomatoes, and cucumbers
  - Activity: 20-minute walk during lunch break
- Evening:
  - Dinner: Grilled shrimp with whole grain pasta and a side of asparagus
  - Activity: Light relaxation exercises

Thursday:
- Morning:
  - Exercise: 30-minute strength training
  - Breakfast: Whole-grain toast with avocado and a poached egg
- Afternoon:
  - Lunch: Lentil soup with a whole grain roll
  - Activity: 10-minute progressive muscle relaxation
- Evening:
  - Dinner: Chicken stir-fry with a variety of vegetables
  - Activity: 10-minute meditation

Friday:
- Morning:
  - Exercise: 30-minute light jog
  - Breakfast: Scrambled eggs with spinach and tomatoes
- Afternoon:
  - Lunch: Tuna salad with mixed greens and a vinaigrette dressing

 - Activity: 20-minute social activity (call a friend or family member)
- Evening:
 - Dinner: Baked cod with sweet potatoes and green beans
 - Activity: Reflective journaling about the week's positive experiences

Saturday:
- Morning:
 - Exercise: 1-hour dance class or fun activity like hiking
 - Breakfast: Pancakes made with whole grains and topped with fresh fruit
- Afternoon:
 - Lunch: Veggie wrap with hummus and a side of carrot sticks
 - Activity: Outdoor activity or hobby (gardening, painting)
- Evening:
 - Dinner: Grilled steak with a side of roasted vegetables
 - Activity: 10-minute meditation

Sunday:
- Morning:
 - Exercise: 30-minute yoga session
 - Breakfast: Smoothie bowl with granola and fruits
- Afternoon:
 - Lunch: Baked chicken with mixed greens and a light dressing
 - Activity: Plan healthy meals and activities for the upcoming week
- Evening:
 - Dinner: Vegetable and bean chili with a side of cornbread
 - Activity: Relax with a book or a warm bath

POST-TRAUMATIC STRESS DISORDER (PTSD)

Monday:
- Morning:
  - Exercise: 30-minute brisk walk
  - Breakfast: Smoothie with spinach, banana, almond milk, and protein powder
- Afternoon:
  - Lunch: Quinoa salad with chickpeas, tomatoes, and cucumbers
  - Activity: Body scan meditation (focus on different parts of the body to release tension)
- Evening:
  - Dinner: Baked salmon with quinoa and steamed broccoli
  - Activity: Light yoga session focusing on grounding techniques

Tuesday:
- Morning:
  - Exercise: 45-minute cycling session
  - Breakfast: Greek yogurt with honey and berries
- Afternoon:
  - Lunch: Turkey and avocado wrap with a side of mixed greens
  - Activity: Tension and trauma releasing exercises (TRE)
- Evening:
  - Dinner: Vegetable stir-fry with tofu and brown rice
  - Activity: 10-minute mindfulness meditation

Wednesday:
- Morning:
  - Exercise: 30-minute swimming
  - Breakfast: Smoothie bowl with granola and fruits

- Afternoon:
  - Lunch: Lentil soup with a whole grain roll
  - Activity: Somatic experiencing exercises (focus on physical sensations related to trauma)
- Evening:
  - Dinner: Grilled shrimp with whole grain pasta and a side of asparagus
  - Activity: Light stretching and relaxation exercises

Thursday:
- Morning:
  - Exercise: 30-minute strength training
  - Breakfast: Whole-grain toast with avocado and a poached egg
- Afternoon:
  - Lunch: Tuna salad with mixed greens and a vinaigrette dressing
  - Activity: Grounding exercises (focus on the present moment using the senses)
- Evening:
  - Dinner: Baked cod with sweet potatoes and green beans
  - Activity: Watch a feel-good movie or show

Friday:
- Morning:
  - Exercise: 30-minute light jog
  - Breakfast: Scrambled eggs with spinach and tomatoes
- Afternoon:
  - Lunch: Veggie wrap with hummus and a side of carrot sticks
  - Activity: Progressive muscle relaxation (PMR)
- Evening:
  - Dinner: Grilled steak with a side of roasted vegetables

- Activity: Reflective journaling about positive experiences of the week

Saturday:
- Morning:
  - Exercise: 1-hour dance class or fun activity like hiking
  - Breakfast: Pancakes made with whole grains and topped with fresh fruit
- Afternoon:
  - Lunch: Quinoa salad with chickpeas, tomatoes, and cucumbers
  - Activity: Art therapy (drawing or painting emotions and experiences)
- Evening:
  - Dinner: Chicken stir-fry with a variety of vegetables
  - Activity: Gentle stretching and relaxation exercises

Sunday:
- Morning:
  - Exercise: 30-minute yoga session
  - Breakfast: Smoothie bowl with granola and fruits
- Afternoon:
  - Lunch: Baked chicken with mixed greens and a light dressing
  - Activity: Plan meals and activities for the upcoming week
- Evening:
  - Dinner: Vegetable and bean chili with a side of cornbread
  - Activity: Relax with a book or a warm bath

DEPRESSION

Monday:
- Morning:
  - Exercise: 30-minute brisk walk in nature
  - Breakfast: Oatmeal with berries and nuts
- Afternoon:
  - Lunch: Grilled chicken salad with a variety of vegetables
  - Activity: 15-minute journaling about feelings and thoughts
- Evening:
  - Dinner: Baked salmon with quinoa and steamed broccoli
  - Activity: Gentle yoga session focusing on relaxation

Tuesday:
- Morning:
  - Exercise: 45-minute cycling session
  - Breakfast: Greek yogurt with honey and berries
- Afternoon:
  - Lunch: Turkey and avocado wrap with a side of mixed greens
  - Activity: Engage in a creative activity (drawing, painting)
- Evening:
  - Dinner: Vegetable stir-fry with tofu and brown rice
  - Activity: 10-minute mindfulness meditation

Wednesday:
- Morning:
  - Exercise: 30-minute swimming
  - Breakfast: Smoothie with spinach, banana, almond milk, and protein powder
- Afternoon:
  - Lunch: Quinoa salad with chickpeas, tomatoes, and cucumbers

- Activity: Social activity (call a friend, attend a support group)
- Evening:
 - Dinner: Grilled shrimp with whole grain pasta and a side of asparagus
 - Activity: Light stretching and relaxation exercises

Thursday:
- Morning:
 - Exercise: 30-minute strength training
 - Breakfast: Whole-grain toast with avocado and a poached egg
- Afternoon:
 - Lunch: Lentil soup with a whole grain roll
 - Activity: Practice deep breathing exercises
- Evening:
 - Dinner: Chicken stir-fry with a variety of vegetables
 - Activity: Watch a feel-good movie or show

Friday:
- Morning:
 - Exercise: 30-minute light jog
 - Breakfast: Scrambled eggs with spinach and tomatoes
- Afternoon:
 - Lunch: Tuna salad with mixed greens and a vinaigrette dressing
 - Activity: Spend time on a hobby (gardening, knitting)
- Evening:
 - Dinner: Baked cod with sweet potatoes and green beans
 - Activity: Reflective journaling about positive experiences of the week

Saturday:
- Morning:

- Exercise: 1-hour dance class or fun activity like hiking
- Breakfast: Pancakes made with whole grains and topped with fresh fruit
- Afternoon:
- Lunch: Veggie wrap with hummus and a side of carrot sticks
- Activity: Volunteer or help someone in need
- Evening:
- Dinner: Grilled steak with a side of roasted vegetables
- Activity: Gentle stretching and relaxation exercises

Sunday:
- Morning:
- Exercise: 30-minute yoga session
- Breakfast: Smoothie bowl with granola and fruits
- Afternoon:
- Lunch: Baked chicken with mixed greens and a light dressing
- Activity: Plan meals and activities for the upcoming week
- Evening:
- Dinner: Vegetable and bean chili with a side of cornbread
- Activity: Relax with a book or a warm bath

RAPED WOMEN

Monday:
- Morning:
- Exercise: 30-minute gentle walk in a safe and quiet environment
- Breakfast: Smoothie with spinach, banana, almond milk, and protein powder
- Afternoon:

- Lunch: Quinoa salad with chickpeas, tomatoes, and cucumbers
  - Activity: Breath practice focusing on deep and slow breathing to promote relaxation
- Evening:
  - Dinner: Baked salmon with quinoa and steamed broccoli
  - Activity: Light yoga session focusing on grounding techniques

Tuesday:
- Morning:
  - Exercise: 45-minute cycling session
  - Breakfast: Greek yogurt with honey and berries
- Afternoon:
  - Lunch: Turkey and avocado wrap with a side of mixed greens
  - Activity: Trauma Releasing Exercises (TRE) to release physical tension healing-the-
- Evening:
  - Dinner: Vegetable stir-fry with tofu and brown rice
  - Activity: 10-minute mindfulness meditation

Wednesday:
- Morning:
  - Exercise: 30-minute swimming
  - Breakfast: Smoothie bowl with granola and fruits
- Afternoon:
  - Lunch: Lentil soup with a whole grain roll
  - Activity: Body scan meditation to increase body awareness and release tension
- Evening:
  - Dinner: Grilled shrimp with whole grain pasta and a side of asparagus

- Activity: Light stretching and relaxation exercises sexual-trauma.

Thursday:
- Morning:
  - Exercise: 30-minute strength training
  - Breakfast: Whole-grain toast with avocado and a poached egg
- Afternoon:
  - Lunch: Tuna salad with mixed greens and a vinaigrette dressing
  - Activity: Grounding exercises using sensory focus to stay present healing-the-sacred-
- Evening:
  - Dinner: Baked cod with sweet potatoes and green beans
  - Activity: Watch a feel-good movie or show

Friday:
- Morning:
  - Exercise: 30-minute light jog
  - Breakfast: Scrambled eggs with spinach and tomatoes
- Afternoon:
  - Lunch: Veggie wrap with hummus and a side of carrot sticks
  - Activity: Progressive muscle relaxation (PMR) to reduce tension sexual-trauma.htm)]
- Evening:
  - Dinner: Grilled steak with a side of roasted vegetables
  - Activity: Reflective journaling about positive experiences of the week

Saturday:
- Morning:
  - Exercise: 1-hour dance class or fun activity like hiking

- Breakfast: Pancakes made with whole grains and topped with fresh fruit
- Afternoon:
  - Lunch: Quinoa salad with chickpeas, tomatoes, and cucumbers
- Evening:
  - Dinner: Chicken stir-fry with a variety of vegetables
  - Activity: Gentle stretching and relaxation exercises

Sunday:
- Morning:
  - Exercise: 30-minute yoga session
  - Breakfast: Smoothie bowl with granola and fruits
- Afternoon:
  - Lunch: Baked chicken with mixed greens and a light dressing
  - Activity: Plan meals and activities for the upcoming week
- Evening:
  - Dinner: Vegetable and bean chili with a side of cornbread
  - Activity: Relax with a book or a warm bath.

THE END